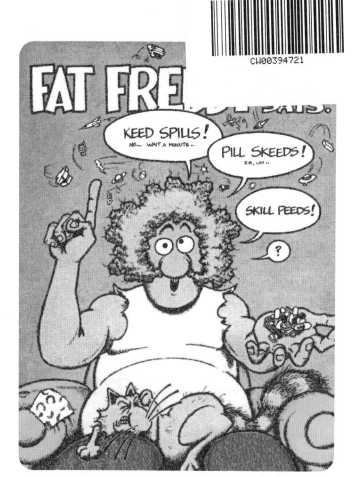

Above: Advice from an expert. Image from Fat Freddy's Cat.
Illustration © Gilbert Shelton, courtesy Knockabout Comics.

First published 2020
© Wooden Books Ltd 2020

Published by Wooden Books Ltd.
Glastonbury, Somerset

British Library Cataloguing in Publication Data
Sessa, B.
Altered States

A CIP catalogue record for this book
may be obtained from the British Library

ISBN-10: 1-904263-85-2
ISBN-13: 978-1-904263-85-2

Designed and typeset in Glastonbury, UK.

Printed in China on 100% FSC
approved sustainable papers by FSC
RR Donnelley Asia Printing Solutions Ltd.

ALTERED STATES
MINDS, DRUGS AND CULTURE

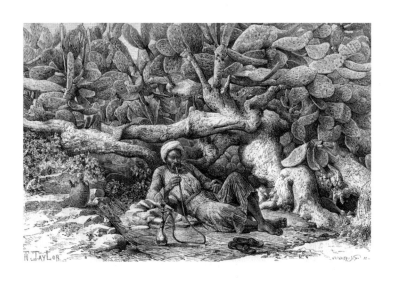

Dr. Ben Sessa

This book is dedicated to those unfortunate people who have been denied access to safe and efficacious medicines, those worthy psychonauts criminalised for pushing the boundaries of senseless laws and to the courageous clinicians and policy makers who are making a stand against the greatest socio-political folly of modern times. The War on Drugs is almost over. The future looks bright. Thanks to the team at Wooden Books, especially Matt Tweed for his editorial assistance and excellent drawings of the neurochemistry and various molecules in the book.

Disclaimer: The author and the publisher accept no responsibility for the misuse of any information in this book, which is intended solely to educate its readers. If you are experimenting with drugs we strongly advise you to read up on the risks, safe doses, side effects and incompatibilities with known medical conditions, just as you would before, say, going mountain climbing, bungie jumping or scuba diving.

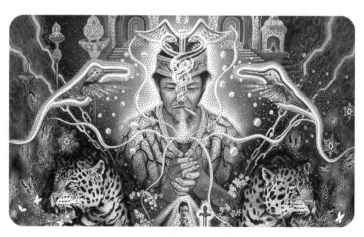

Title page: Man smoking a hookah by a cactus hedge in Jenin, Israel, c.1885, via Shutterstock. Above: Ayahuasca vision, after a painting by Juan Taminchi.

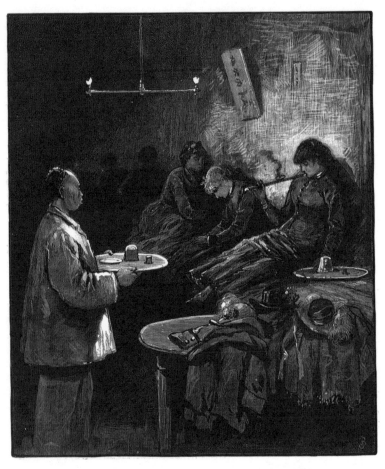

Above: "A Growing Metropolitan Evil. Scene in an opium den in Pell Street,
frequented by working girls." From sketches by C. Upham, London, c.1911.

INTRODUCTION

IN THE SAME WAY that common consciousness is integral to human experience, so too are our altered states. Beyond the trappings of our civilised version of humanity, few of us have ever been wholly content with everyday waking awareness, not when we have the capacity to seek, recognise and experience alternative states of consciousness, and see the day from a slightly different angle.

There are so many ways to alter our consciousness, from music, drugs and our choice of food to meditation, dance and exercise. Because and perhaps in spite of this, attempts to expand consciousness have been both worshipped and demonised throughout human history. For example, just being inside a church, with its subdued light, etherial voices and reverent atmosphere, can encourage the free association of other-worldly feelings, and that is before you drink any holy wine. Other religions owe their origins to the archaic use of hallucinogenic plants and fungi. All seek a magnificent glimpse of the oceanic boundlessness that seems to exist just beyond our usual awareness—an altered state of consciousness,

Our passion for altered states may also have given us evolutionary advantage over less sentient species. It is perhaps a privilege of the human condition, with its lofty claims of spirituality and consciousness, that we reserve the right to alter it. After all, one man's cognitive impairment is another man's party and we have, it seems, become masters and mistresses of messing with the brain and her tenuous attempts to remain straight.

So, welcome to this journey into the hinterlands of consciousness expansion. Along the way we will encounter pounding hearts, cosmic sex, smouldering herbs and psychedelic potatoes. Not to mention a pinch or two of phanerothyme.

STATES OF CONSCIOUSNESS
intentional and unintentional

MOST OF THE TIME, most of us, when we are awake, sober, in good health and not spiritually enlightened, experience NORMAL CLEAR CONSCIOUSNESS— we know *where* we are, *when* we are and (crucially) *who* we are. Psychiatrists call this being ORIENTATED IN TIME, PLACE & PERSON.

In an altered state, however, the qualitative experience of consciousness is different. Perceptions change, and one may feel disorientated. This is described formally as a DELIRIUM or an ACUTE CONFUSIONAL STATE.

Consciousness may be altered intentionally, accidentally or as part of normal life, such as SLEEP and DREAMING (*p.10*). Intentional causes include FASTING (*p.22*), EXERCISE (*p.16*), HYPERVENTILATION (*p.16*), SENSORY DEPRIVATION (*opposite*), STIMULATION with lights and sounds and the ingestion of psychoactive DRUGS (*pp.34-51*). Non-intentional causes include TRAUMA and DEPRIVATION (e.g. head or brain injuries, and starvation) or DISEASE (e.g. fevers and epilepsy). Any of these can affect usual functioning and produce hallucinations and other psychiatric symptoms.

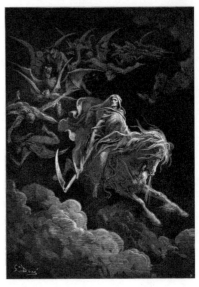

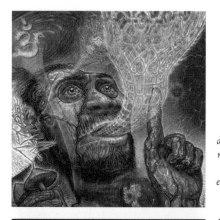

Left: **MAGIC MUSHROOMS**, by Alex Grey. Modern humans only appeared in the last 200,000 years. **PSILOCYBIN** (see page 46) increases visual acuity, giving mushroom-eaters an evolutionary advantage. Perhaps early hominids, with senses heightened from psychedelic fungi growing on cow dung, developed their external & internal dialogue to make sense of their new and interesting stream of consciousness. Language would also have enabled the understanding of complex concepts and internal representations of the world.

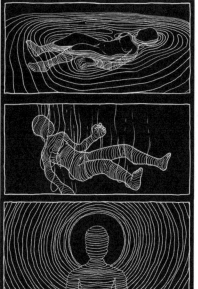

Left: **SENSORY DEPRIVATION TANK**, by Luke Howard. An absence of sensory perceptions will trigger an altered state in an awake brain (e.g. hallucinations in prisoners or prophets in solitary confinement). In 1954, American neuroscientist John Lilly built a lightless, soundproof tank inside which a person could float effortlessly in salt water at skin temperature. Devoid of touch, sound and sight, subjects often reported unusual experiences. Instead of sleeping, the brain fills in the gaps, using its stores of memories and imagary to bombard the floater with sensory experiences and colourful visions. Users also reported an intense experience of deep relaxation that had lasting, healing, mystical and spiritual consequences. Floatation tanks are used to relieve anxiety disorders, chronic pain, depression and a wide range of addictions.

Facing page: Vision of Death, engraving by Gustav Doré, 1868.

3

THE BRAIN
neurons and networks

The brain has been viewed in many ways—as an engine, a soul, even as food. The body's primary computer, it regulates multiple complex processes, including a mechanism for appreciating consciousness itself.

Biologically, the brain is a network of specialized cells, called *neurons*. Nearly 90 billion neurons connect via long *axons*, which can each branch into thousands of *telodendria* which then connect to the shorter local receptive *dendrites* of other neurons. Nerve messages from neurons are sent down the axons as electrical *action potentials*. On reaching a *synapse*, where an *axon terminal* of one neuron meets a dendritic receptor of another neuron, the potential triggers the release of *neurotransmitter* chemicals which cross the narrow synaptic gap and bind to receptors on the dendrite.

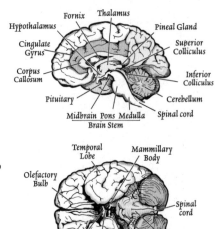

Some neurotransmitters and some receptors *inhibit* neuron activity, while others *excite* the action. The input from up to 7,000 dendrites is then tallied up inside each neuron and the new action potential sent out, down its axon and axon branches, all of this influencing, much further downstream, your eventual mental experience.

4

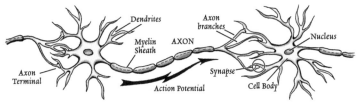

Above: Two connected **NEURONS**. *Neurons collect information via their short dendrites and adjust their rate of fire accordingly, which is then transmitted down their long axon and its branches to other neurons.*

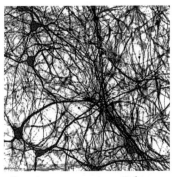

Above: A **NEURAL NETWORK**. *Each neuron can have up to 7,000 dendrons. There are c. 100 trillion neural connections in a human brain.*

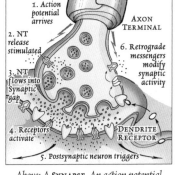

Above: A **SYNAPSE**. *An action potential arrives, releasing neurotransmitters (NT) which excite or inhibit the next neuron firing.*

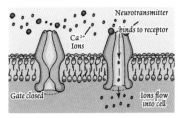

Above: **IONOTROPIC RECEPTORS** *form gates in cell membranes. When open, increased ion concentration causes the cell to trigger.*

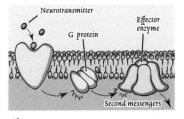

Above: **METABOTROPIC RECEPTORS** *act on G proteins, causing effector enzymes to send second messengers to alter cell function.*

NEUROTRANSMITTERS
and hormones

Our brains use over 100 neurotransmitters, some small molecules, others larger proteins. GLUTAMATE, the most common, is excitatory, whereas GAMMA-AMINOBUTYRIC ACID (GABA) conversely is inhibitory (depressant drugs like alcohol (*p.30*) and benzodiazepines (*p.10*) work by mimicking GABA). DOPAMINE (*below*) is central to motor behaviour activities, and pleasure and reward processes. SEROTONIN, mostly made in the intestine, regulates sleep, memory, appetite, learning and mood. NOREPINEPHRINE moderates sleep patterns, focus and alertness. EPINEPHRINE, released from the adrenal glands, helps us to stay alert and is intrinsic to the fear-stimulated fight-flight-freeze response. HISTAMINE is involved in local immune responses, including itching and inflammation.

Hormones work alongside neurotransmitters. Over 100 of these chemical messengers of the endocrine system are produced in organs throughout the body, including the heart, thyroid, kidneys, gonads, liver and pancreas. Hormones have a broad regulatory effect on physiological functioning and also act on the brain, particularly the pituitary gland (*opposite top*), which secretes hormones to regulate the output of other hormones in the body that control our overall metabolism and levels of hunger, thirst, libido, stress, joy and growth. All of these in turn affect our state of mind.

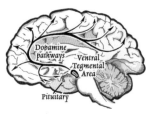

DOPAMINE $C_8H_{11}NO_2$

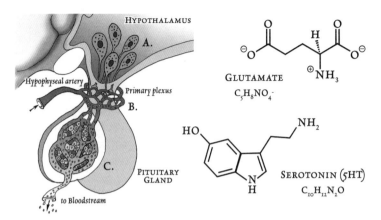

Above left: Neuroendocrine cell bodies [A] make Corticotropin Releasing Factor (CRF) in the Hypothalamus, which passes to the pituitary via the Primary Plexus [B]. Hormone-producing cells [C] release Adreno-corticotropic hormone (ACTH) and β-endorphin to regulate further endocrine glands across the body.

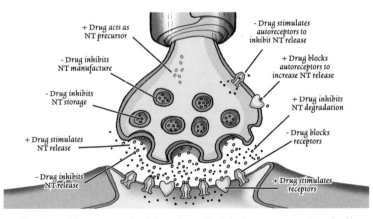

Above: Some of the many ways that different drugs affect the brain via neurotransmitters (NT). Facing page: Dopamine pathways include the Mesocorticolimbic projection (shown) which is associated with reward-related cognition, incentive salience (wanting), pleasure (liking) and other processes.

Oxytocin & Adrenaline
romance and other horrors

From the myriad of factors that create our emotional lives, two hormones in particular, *oxytocin* and *adrenaline*, shape our experience of love and fear.

OXYTOCIN, the "love hormone", is released by women more than men during and after sex and is also present during childbirth and breastfeeding. It induces feelings of empathy, sexual bonding and relationship-building, resulting in increased prosocial behaviour and sensitivity to certain socially relevant stimuli. Produced in the pituitary gland, deep within the brain, it also soothes the *amygdala*, part of the ancient *limbic system* in the centre of the brain, which mediates emotions, particularly the fear response.

ADRENALINE (*epinephrine*), "the fear hormone", is secreted from a gland on top of the kidney, (*ad* 'on top of', *renal* 'kidney'), and from neurons in the *medulla oblongata* in the brain. It is governed by signals from the autonomic nervous system, particularly those triggered by fear, mediated by the amygdala. It plays an important role in the fight-flight-freeze response by increasing blood sugar levels, boosting the output of the heart, increasing blood flow to the muscles and causing pupil dilation—allowing the organism to either stand and fight, run away or freeze and play dead. Thus the concept of the 'adrenaline junkie', who enjoys thrill-seeking behaviour, including extreme sports and risk-taking activities such as substance abuse, crime and unsafe sex.

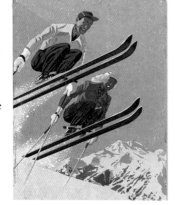

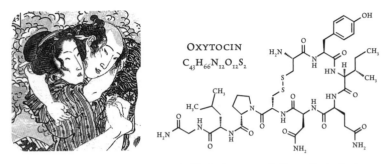

OXYTOCIN

$C_{43}H_{66}N_{12}O_{12}S_2$

Above: **OXYTOCIN.** *Many activities increase blood levels of oxytocin, including meditating, having an orgasm or a hot bath, petting animals and hugging. It is also increased by certain drugs, notably MDMA and Viagra. Clinically it has been explored as an antidepressant and an anti-addictive, as it appears to inhibit tolerance to some addictive drugs, including alcohol, opiates and cocaine.*

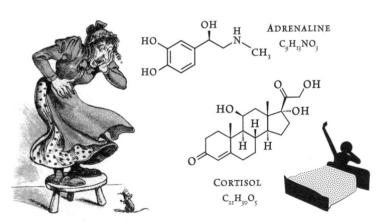

ADRENALINE

$C_9H_{13}NO_3$

CORTISOL

$C_{21}H_{30}O_5$

Above left: **ADRENALINE** *and* **CORTISOL** *"the wakeup hormone." Both are produced in the adrenal gland and increase blood sugar. However cortisol, a steroid hormone, is also produced at other times, on a diurnal cycle, being released in large amounts on waking in the morning, then dropping throughout the day. It aids the metabolism of protein, fat and carbohydrates and inhibits bone formation.*

DREAMING
sleep and sleeping pills

DREAMING is undoubtedly the most common altered state in humans. Almost everyone dreams. However, it remains a mysterious phenomenon, begging questions as to how consciousness relates to the world.

The physiology of dreaming involves changing electrical activity in the brain (*see opposite top*). During dreaming, the eyeballs flicker under the lids, as if scanning the waking world. Strangely, dreamers are mostly unaware that they are dreaming, simply accepting the peculiar scenarios.

There are instances of **LUCID DREAMING**, in which the dreamer manipulates the dream, taking themselves on wilful journeys of fantasy. Some people enhance this experience with **GALANTAMINE** or **CALEA ZACATECHICHI**, a plant long used by the Chontal Indians of Mexico.

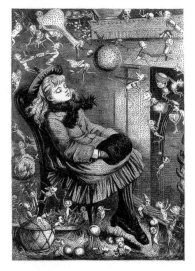

BARBITURATES were used as sleeping pills from c. 1900–1960. Today, these have been replaced by **BENZODIAZEPINES** (e.g. **DIAZEPAM**, **LORAZEPAM** and **NITRAZEPAM**) and **Z-DRUGS** (e.g. **ZOPICLONE** and **ZOLPIDEM**). Both types activate the GABA (inhibitory) system, shorten the time spent falling asleep, prolong the sleep time and reduce wakefulness. All create significant dependence affects and generally ought not to be taken long term.

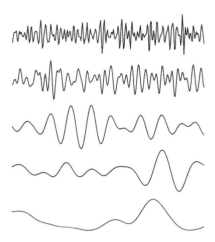

GAMMA WAVES   120 − 31 hz
rapid brain activity, deep learning

BETA WAVES   30 − 13 hz
normal waking state

ALPHA WAVES   12 - 8 hz
relaxed, meditative

THETA WAVES   7 − 4 hz
drowsy, nodding off, dreaming

DELTA WAVES   3 − 0.5 hz
dreamless sleep

Above: **BRAIN WAVES:** *Awake gamma and beta brain waves pulse from 120–13 hertz. Closing the eyes and relaxing slows the waves to an alpha band of 12–8 hz. Drowsier still and the rate drops to the theta band at 7–4 hz, then to delta deep of up to 3 hz. The sleeper finally enters* **RAPID EYE MOVEMENT** *(REM) sleep, where dreams occur and the brain appears lively, almost as if awake.*

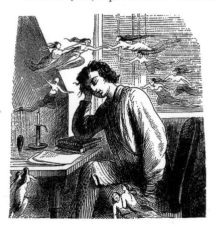

Left: The bizarre relevance of **DREAMS** *to wishes and fears strongly indicates that dreaming accesses the unconscious mind. As dreams often develop without external stimuli, it seems they come from internal transformations of stored material. They may be swamped with symbolism, making dream interpretation a popular and sometimes potent activity through history. During sleep, supplies of* **ADENOSINE TRIPHOSPHATE** *(ATP), the molecule used for short-term storage and transport of energy, are replenished, and growth hormone and prolactin are released.*

HYPNOTIC STATES
trance and suggestibility

The brain's ability to create and respond to imagery (as in dreams) is exploited in **TRANCE** states by therapists, storytellers, DJs and advertisers. Different individuals experience trance in different ways. Some easily daydream and use reverie to solve problems, while for others the trance state is very different from their waking consciousness.

During **HYPNOSIS**, EEGs of subjects show mainly beta wave activity, with some mild alpha waves, suggestive of light sleep. Most people remain awake, so hypnosis is not a unitary state of consciousness, rather there are fluctuations in brain activity. Subjects tend to be hyper-relaxed and able to focus intensely as directed, following suggestions while disassociated from external distractions. In clinical practice these features have been utilised in **HYPNOTHERAPY**, helping with conditions like depression, anxiety, eating disorders, PTSD, smoking and obesity. Hypnosis causes a decrease in activity in the *dorsal anterior cingulate*, which results in reduced rumination and worrying. There is also a disconnect between one's actions and one's awareness of one's actions.

Some other techniques (*e.g. see opposite*) prevent a drift into delta sleep, which keeps subjects in the theta stage, inducing a **HYPNOGOGIC STATE** of non-ordinary consciousness. This can allow access to aspects of personal psychology and core personality that may otherwise remain veiled.

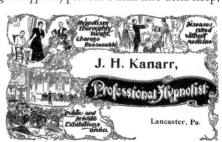

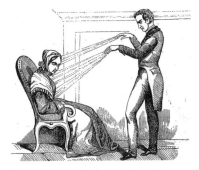

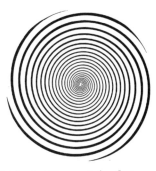

Above: **MESMERISM.** *In the 1770s, Franz Mesmer postulated an invisible magnetic force flowing through the body. In 1842, Scottish surgeon James Braid coined the term "hypnosis" (sleep). The 19th C. neurologist Jean-Martin Charcot used hypnotism to treat hysteria, as did his student, Sigmund Freud.*

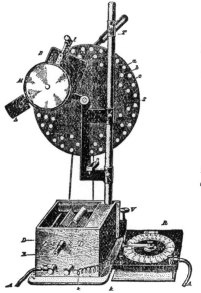

Left: A **STROBOSCOPE,** *a 19th century device for creating flashing lights which can produce altered states of consciousness in some people. The process of* **LOGOTHERAPY** *uses a stroboscope with variable speeds and intensity combined with a constant light source to purportedly activate different types of bodily and mental experiences.*

SOUNDS *too can also alter consciousness.* **BINAURAL BEATS,** *a process discovered by 19th century physicist Heinrich Wilhelm Dove, entails listening to two separate tones presented at slightly different frequencies – one to each ear. The sounds mix together slightly out of sync and produce a low-frequency pulsation. Improvements in sleep and learning have been reported as well as profound out-of-body experiences, astral projection and telepathy.*

MEDITATION
quieting the mind

MEDITATION is as old as the mind itself. The foundations of Buddhism and Hinduism revolve around the practice of tranquility, of transcendental connectivity with the other through the stillness of the self. In this altered state the meditator develops compassion by refining their own awareness.

Regular meditators have been shown to have better immune responses, more stable blood pressure and lower respiratory rates. Studies have demonstrated decreased activity in the amygdala (*see page 8*), which correlates to reduced self-reported stress levels. Some types of meditation reduce activity in the sympathetic nervous system and increase activity in the parasympathetic nervous system. Further evidence suggests the medial prefrontal cortex and the posterior cingulate cortex become relatively deactivated during meditation.

In some cultures individuals meditate alone, in others they meditate together. Some use silent breath, others music, chanting, laughter, tears, movement or sex. One thing all practices have in common is the altered state of consciousness that underpins the therapeutic and healing effects of meditation. Meditation remains the oldest and surest way of living life in a permanently altered state of consciousness.

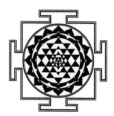
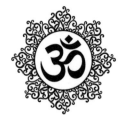
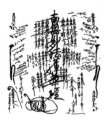

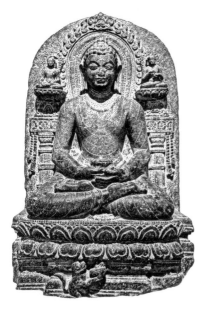

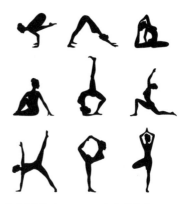

Left: Meditating BUDDHA, India, Pala dynasty, c.1000AD. Above: YOGA was developed to aid long periods of motionless meditation. Facing page, left to right: SRI YANTRA; sacred OM sign; Namu Myōhō Renge Kyō, the mantra of Nichiren Buddhism. Below: Table of MEDITATIONS.

MEDITATION TYPE	FOCUS ON	EXAMPLES
SOUND	wind, running water, chimes, singing bowls, birds, silence	SHAMANIC DRUMMING, SOUND MEDITATIONS
VISUALISATION	point of light, loved one, colour, clouds, leaves, guided journey, inner landscape	PRAYER, COLOUR HEALING, AFFIRMATION
MOVEMENT	muscle flow, changing shape, balance, stillness in motion, breathing while moving	YOGA, TAI CHI, QI GONG, WALK/JOGGING, DANCE
REPETITION	repeated mantra, question e.g. 'who am I', breath counting, chanting, movement	MANTRA, CHANT, KIRTAN, FASTING,
BREATH	on turning of breath, holding of breath, length of breath, quality of breath	BUDDHIST, VEDIC, YOGIC, HAWAIAN
SELF-OBSERVATION	emotions, life purpose, addictions, relationships, heart, body scan	PURE AWARENESS, CONTEMPLATION,
MINDFULNESS	on nature of self, I-other dichotomy, unity, sensory illusion, cosmos	ZEN, VIPASSANA, CH'AN, NON-DUALITY

15

ENDORPHINS
run rabbit run

Pleasurable activities like SEX, EXERCISE and EATING cause the pituitary and hypothalamus glands to secrete the body's own endogenous MORPHINES (*p.42*), the ENDORPHINS. These, along with SEROTONIN (*p.6*), ADRENALINE (*p.8*) and ENDOCANNABINOIDS (*p.34*), which are also secreted during exercise, lead to feelings of euphoria, an enhanced immune response and the release of sex hormones. Many people work out not only to be healthier, but also to feel more alive and high—thus the long history of humans pushing themselves to the limit to gain altered states.

Endorphins are also released in response to tissue damage, acting as an analgesic, bringing relief from pain. This makes evolutionary sense, as breaking through the pain barrier must have given early humans an advantage when hunting. Endorphins are neurotransmitters, and reduce pain by interacting with opiate receptors in the brain, similarly to drugs such as morphine and codeine. This may explain why excessive exercise and intentional self-harm can be addictive; indeed, some treatments for self-harmers use an opiate blocker to quell the reward feelings of endorphins.

Extreme HYPERVENTILATION may also be harnessed to enter an altered state. Certain types of breathwork utilise fast deep breathing with music and bodywork to achieve personal growth and spiritual development.

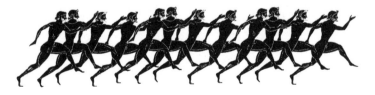

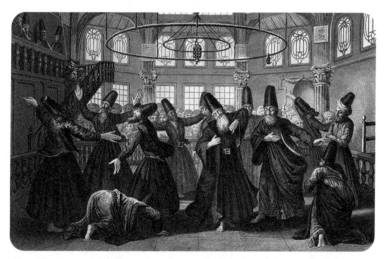

β-ENDORPHIN

$C_{158}H_{251}N_{39}O_{46}S$

Above: **BETA ENDORPHIN**. *Endorphins are naturally occurring endogenous morphine-like chemicals that decrease feelings of pain and are released throughout the body in response to the experience of pain. They also enhance the immune response, provide feelings of euphoria, and release sex hormones.*

Above: The **SUFI WHIRLING DERVISHES** *induce an endorphin-rich trance (see too page 12), by spinning for hours, mirroring the dance of earth and sun. The ancient Indian art of yoga combines endorphin-producing physical, mental and spiritual practices to reach a state of liberation. Meditation, part of the Tibetan tradition, triggers the release of endorphins and increases dopamine, serotonin and melatonin.*

Sex & Aphrodisiacs
euphoric kundalini

From a neurobiological perspective, **SEX** is perhaps the most pleasurable human experience, producing a delirious transcendental state. Throughout history it has been used as a vehicle to commune not only with a partner but also with higher powers. **TANTRIC SEX** (*see opposite*) elevates the mental state so that physical, sexual, emotional and spiritual aspects merge, the ego dissolves and a peak state of sexual ecstasy is maintained.

In males, stimulation of the erect penis results in decreases in blood flow to the right amygdala, which results in a reduction in anxiety. During ejaculation, there is an increase in blood flow to the cerebellum and a stimulation of the brain's reward system. In females, orgasm activates the prefrontal cortex, the orbitofrontal cortex, the insula, the cingulate gyrus and the cerebellum—all of which are involved in the processing of emotions, the sensation of pain and decision-making.

Sexual pleasure provides evolutionary advantage, suggesting that altered consciousness itself may also have evolutionary benefit. Being "out of one's head" is akin to being at the point of sexual ecstasy—a desirable mental state worth seeking out and repeating. There is also a smorgasbord of drugs which purport to enhance sex (*see opposite*), though as Shakespeare noted of alcohol, some *provoketh the desire but taketh away the performance.*

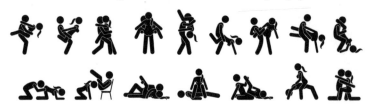

18

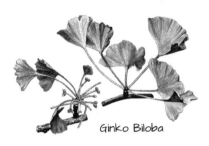

Ginko Biloba

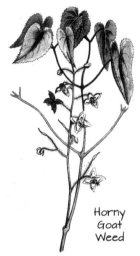

Horny
Goat
Weed

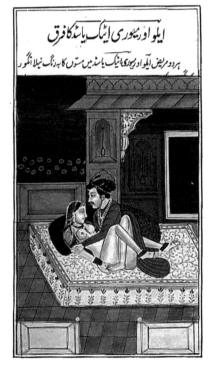

Above: Two **Aphrodisiacs** *used for love
potions to aid sexual ecstasy. Others include*
**Ginseng, Spanish Fly, Watermelon,
Deer Musk** *and* **Oysters.** *Other
popular recreational drugs for enhancing
sexual pleasure include* **Amphetamine,
methamphetamine** *and* **MDMA** *(p.44),*
Cannabis *(p.34),* **Alkyl Nitrates**
(poppers, see p.37) and **GHB.**

*Left: 19th century painting from an Indian
Kama Sutra.* **Tantric Sex** *derives from
traditional Indian Buddhist practice.*
Neotantra *hones the Kundalini energies
that emerge during sex, and uses special
techniques to augment the experience.*

Facing page: 16 different sex positions.

EMOTIONAL STATES
hormones and moods

Everyone experiences dramatic changes in emotion—we can all become fearful, angry or frustrated within moments of feeling happy or elated.

Many conditions and lifestyle choices can cause severe mood changes. In men, high levels of **TESTOSTERONE** and **STEROIDS** are associated with raised levels of anger, aggression, mood swings, hypomania, irritability and depressive episodes. In women, Premenstrual Syndrome (PMS) is a group of symptoms that occur 1–2 weeks before a period, the most likely reason being shifting oestrogen levels. In the days and weeks before a period, a woman's oestrogen levels rise and fall dramatically, levelling out 1 to 2 days after menstruation begins. Around 90% of women experience some PMS symptoms before their periods, the severity varying. Although PMS can cause fatigue, changes in appetite, depression, bloating, and more, it has been overpathologised by male doctors. Premenstrual dysphoric disorder (PMDD) is a more severe and rare type of PMS, found in up to 5% of women of childbearing age. Symptoms of PMDD include sudden shifts in mood, severe depression, extreme irritability, and more.

At menopause, some women experience changes in mood, hot flushes, insomnia and reduced sex drive. This is often over-treated with *hormone replacement therapy* (HRT), which can also help prevent osteoporosis and heart disease. Healthy lifestyle treatments such as avoiding **CAFFEINE** (*p.28*) and **NICOTINE** (*p.32*), geting plenty of **EXERCISE** (*p.16*) and consuming less **ALCOHOL** (*p.30*) and **SUGAR** (*p.24*) can also help to stabilize mood.

   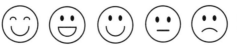

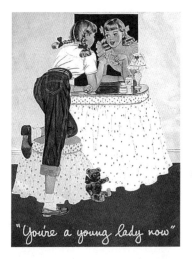

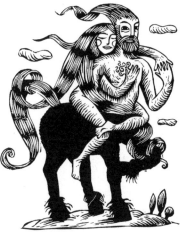

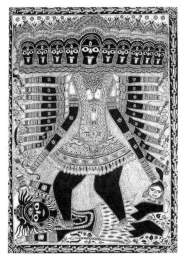

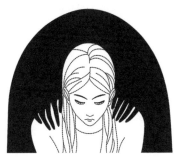

Top left: 1950s advertisment. Top right: Indian woodblock print, c.1990. Left: The Hindu goddess Kali, traditionally shown standing on her consort Shiva and holding a sword and a severed head. Although altered emotional states are not altered states of consciousness, they can often feel like it.

FOOD & FASTING
smells so lovely

Food, and the lack of it, can hugely affect our mental state. For example, OMEGA-3 fatty acids can prevent depression. They occur in OILY FISH, RASPBERRIES, KIWI FRUIT, LINSEED and CANNABIS, although none of these are as good as eating brain itself—some of the highest concentrations are found in mammalian BRAINS and EYES. Other fruits that help with depression include PAPAYA, BANANAS, STRAWBERRIES, MANGOS, PINEAPPLE, GRAPEFRUIT, GUAVA, APRICOTS, PEACHES, APPLES and DATES.

Our sense of smell is also crucial. A smell can trigger desire, disgust or the recall of a long-forgotten experience. Odorous molecules trigger electrical signals that travel to the *olfactory bulb*, a part of the brain's limbic system (hence the close links between smells and emotions). Many animals, particularly insects, communicate via 'smell' using airborne hormones called PHEROMONES. In humans, ANDROSTADIENONE (in male sweat and semen) and ESTRATETRAENOL (in female urine) may play a similar role.

Eating nothing for days, or FASTING, can also affect your state. Practioners describe heightened senses, brighter colours and smells, and improved cognitive function. Fasting stimulates the production of a nerve cell protein which plays a critical role in learning and memory.

Many "poisonous" plants are also psych-oactive. Examples include PSILOCYBIN MUSHROOMS (*p.46*) and GREEN POTATOES (*solanine, right*).

SOLANINE
$C_{45}H_{73}NO_{15}$

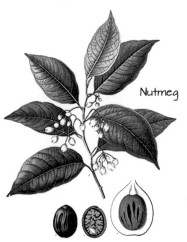

MYRISTICIN
$C_{11}H_{12}O_3$

SAFROLE
$C_{10}H_{10}O_2$

Nutmeg

*Left: Nutmeg's active ingredients **MYRISTICIN**, **ELEMICIN** and **SAFROLE**, are related to the precursors of **MDMA**. However, overeating nutmeg paste produces nausea, flushed skin, bloodshot eyes, dilated pupils, heavy disorientation, motor function impairments, sleep and hallucinations.*

LACTUCIN
$C_{15}H_{16}O_5$

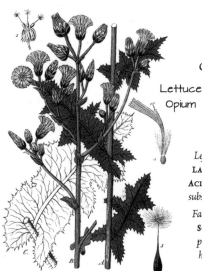

Lettuce Opium

*Left: **LETTUCE OPIUM** contains **LACTUCIN**, **LACTUCEROL** (taraxaxterol) and **LACTUCIC ACID**. It has been used medicinally as an opium substitute and can produce a mild intoxication.*

*Facing page: Raw **GREEN POTATOES** contain **SOLANINE**, a glycoalkaloid which acts as a pesticide and fungicide and can give a mild high as well as vomiting, stomach cramps, headaches and dizziness.*

SUGAR
hide not thy poison

Sugar appears as **FRUCTOSE** and **GLUCOSE** in seasonal fruits and berries, often bonded to form **SUCROSE** (*see opposite*). Through plant breeding and refining humans have become used to high levels of sucrose in both savoury and sweet dishes, despite obesity reaching epidemic proportions.

Eating sugary food primes the *nucleus accumbens* to release **ENDORPHINS** (*p.16*) and **DOPAMINE** (*p.6*), with subsequent euphoric effects. In the body, sucrose is broken back down into fructose and glucose. Glucose as 'blood sugar' is an important source of energy for the body's organs, muscles and nervous system and is regulated by the hormones **INSULIN** and **GLUCAGON** which are produced in the pancreas. Glucose also stimulates both **OPIOID** (*p.42*) and dopamine receptors. Indeed, there are many similarities between drug and sugar addictions, with the same tolerance to high doses, strong cravings and withdrawal symptoms. Genetically, the children of alcoholics demonstrate an abnormally 'sweet tooth'.

The 'sugar rush' is familiar to any parent whose toddler goes wild after eating sugar, though the hyperactivity is more likely due to genetic factors, **CAFFEINE** (*p.28*, in chocolate and drinks) and colouring additives.

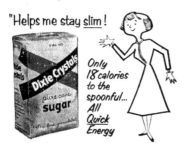

"Helps me stay slim!"

Only 18 calories to the spoonful... All Quick Energy

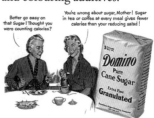

Better go easy on that Sugar! Thought you were counting calories?

You're wrong about sugar, Mother! Sugar in tea or coffee at every meal gives fewer calories than your reducing salad!

It's **smart** to stay slim and trim and get *Domino's* "Energy Lift" too!

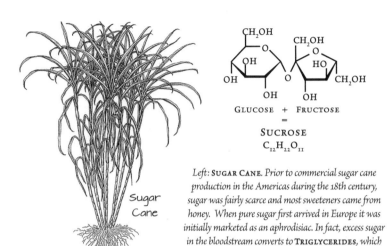

GLUCOSE + FRUCTOSE
=
SUCROSE
$C_{12}H_{22}O_{11}$

Left: SUGAR CANE. Prior to commercial sugar cane production in the Americas during the 18th century, sugar was fairly scarce and most sweeteners came from honey. When pure sugar first arrived in Europe it was initially marketed as an aphrodisiac. In fact, excess sugar in the bloodstream converts to TRIGLYCERIDES, which are stored in more and more fat cells. Not very sexy.

Sugar Cane

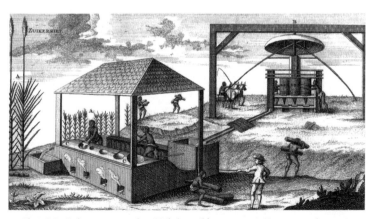

Above: West Indian sugar cane plant. High demand for pure sugar in Europe created a surge in cultivation in the West Indies, driving the slave trade. Production in India pushed the British Empire through the Victorian era, as sugary deserts and chocolate (next page) became essential must-haves.

CHOCOLATE
mayan gold

The earliest recorded use of **CACAO** seeds dates to Central America in 1400 BC, when the Mayans enjoyed them as a bitter alcoholic drink. By the 15th century, the Aztecs had added **VANILLA** and **CHILI PEPPERS**, associated the beverage with the Goddess of fertility and given it the name **XOCOLATI**, from which the word **CHOCOLATE** arises. The Mayan also used cacao beans as a currency, such was the high esteem in which the drink was held.

As well as **SUGAR** (*see p.24*) and **CAFFEINE** (*see p.28*), cacao contains **THEOBROMINE**, a vasodilator and heart stimulant that might be responsible for chocolate's aphrodisiac effects. It also contains **PHENETHYLAMINE**, a natural psychoactive molecule with stimulant properties, closely related to **AMPHETAMINE** and **MDMA** (*see p.44*). Studies suggest chocolate contains significant levels of **ANANDAMIDE**, one of the brain's endogenous **CANNABINOIDS** (*see p.34*), which may add to its euphoric effect. Other studies have shown that whilst eating chocolate, there is observed modulation in cortical chemosensory areas, including the insula and caudomedial and caudolateral OFC, associated with the reward value of food.

Eating chocolate significantly alters our consciousness.

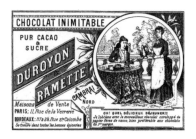

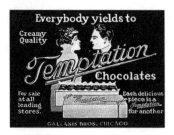

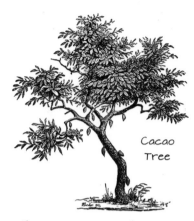

$$\text{PHENETHYLAMINE}$$
$$C_8H_{11}N$$

$$\text{THEOBROMINE}$$
$$C_7H_8N_4O_2$$

Above: **THEOBROMA CACAO**, *the cocoa tree, is a small 4-8m (12-26ft) evergreen tree, native to the tropics of Mesoamerica. Cocoa butter, solids and chocolate are all made from its beans.*

Above: **PHENETHYAMINE** *is a vasodilator and heart stimulant and possible aphrodisiac.* **THEOBROMINE** *is a natural psychoactive. Also active in chocolate is* **ANANDAMIDE.**

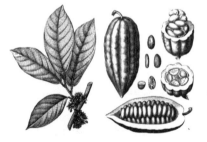

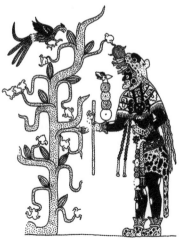

Above: **CACAO PODS.** *Right:* **MAYAN PRIEST** *attending his Cacao plant. Some intrepid chocolate lovers mix large volumes of chocolate with an MAO inhibitor to try and extract the phenethylamine or anandamide – this practice is best avoided unless one wants to precipitate a hypertensive crisis, or Death by Chocolate.*

CAFFEINE
a very nice cup

Some altered states are effective simply because they are not too extreme.

CAFFEINE is a mild stimulant found in a number of plants, particularly in **COFFEE** seeds, **TEA** leaves, **KOLA** nuts and **GUARANA** berries. It can be quite potent and is widely enjoyed. Negative effects include diuresis, insomnia, agitation, palpitations and, in extreme cases, psychosis.

Caffeine keeps you awake in a variety of ways. **ADENOSINE** is a chemical created in the brain that makes you feel tired. Caffeine binds to the brain's adenosine receptors preventing the binding of adenosine. Caffeine also causes blood vessels to dilate, allowing greater blood flow and oxygenation of the brain, which promotes wakefulness. Caffeine also reduces dopamine reabsorption, resulting in raised levels of dopamine and associated feelings of reward and pleasure.

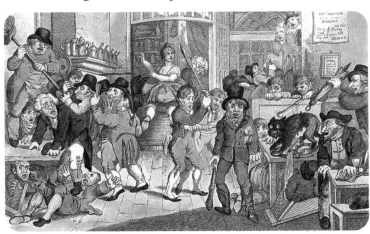

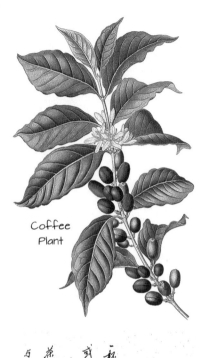

Coffee
Plant

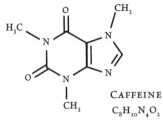

CAFFEINE
$C_8H_{10}N_4O_2$

Above: **CAFFEINE**. *Left: The* **COFFEE PLANT**.
*Facing page: Mad Dog in a Coffee House,
T. Rowlandson, 1809. In the 15th century, coffee
drinking migrated from Sufi monasteries in
Arabia to Europe. By the 17th century, coffee
houses in London, Oxford and Paris were
stimulating debate, spurring on intellectuals
and artists, and curing hangovers along the way.*

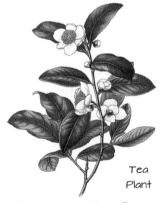

Tea
Plant

Above: **TEA PLANT**. *Tea actually contains
more of the stimulants* **THEOBROMINE** *(p.26)
and* **THEOPHYLLINE** *than caffeine. Left: Tea
drinking dates back 5,000 years to ancient China.*

ALCOHOL
from ginger beer to gin lane

Apart from dreaming, the most familiar altered state for many people is drunkenness—surprising, given how dangerous it is for the health.

ALCOHOLS are organic compounds with an -OH hydroxyl group, but for alcoholic drinks we refer specifically to ETHANOL. Its effect in the body is BIPHASIC, with stimulating early effects in the frontal lobes (the seat of higher function) causing loosened inhibitions, euphoria and relaxation, while later sedative effects kick in as increased dosage reaches the cerebellum, producing slurred speech and motor incoordination. Higher doses effect the brain stem and cause respiratory depression.

Alcohol inhibits anti-diuretic hormones, resulting in diluted urine and dehydration. Heavy frequent drinking leads to physical dependence. Millions of deaths a year are linked to alcohol, along with accidents, assaults, abuse and self-harm. The hangover is due to low blood sugar from alcohol stimulating insulin production.

Alcohol is metabolised in the liver, but with prolonged use this fails and the liver becomes inflamed and scarred which can result in burst vessels and sudden death. Chronic abuse can also lead to liver cancer. Similarly, the heart swells and dies, and the brain packs in. Alcoholic dementia is unfortunately the commonest cause of cognitive impairment in the elderly.

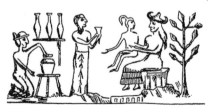
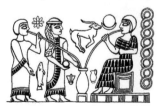

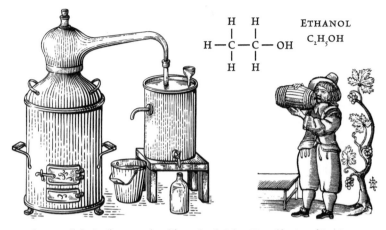

ETHANOL
C₂H₅OH

Above: A still, for distilling pure ethanol from a hooch. Below: Hogarth's prints of Beer Street (wholesome) and Gin Lane (ruinous). Opposite: Egyptian and Mesopotamian murals of beer production, showing that alcohol has been part of human culture for many thousands of years.

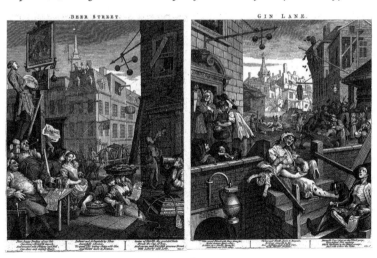

NICOTINE

cigarettes, vapes, snuff and patches

NICOTINE is a potent parasympathetic alkaloid found in several plants, notably in TOBACCO (*Nicotiana tabacum*). Consumption results in the rapid onset of a delicate altered state of consciousness. It is a powerful stimulator of the dopamine-mediated reward system, and is extremely addictive.

Nicotine is absorbed into the bloodstream through the mouth, nose and lungs, acting on endogenous *nicotinic acetylcholine* receptors in the central and sympathetic nervous systems. Effects are generally stimulatory, though there is also a paradoxical relaxation. Anecdotally, smokers say it stimulates the ability to work and socialize, improving confidence and focus.

Obviously, dragging smoke, which contains poisonous chemicals, carbon monoxide and carcinogens, directly into fragile lung tissue is unbelievably bad for health.

Smoking is associated with cardiovascular disease, cancers and birth defects, resulting in over 8m deaths a year worldwide. Pure nicotine, however, is not especially toxic at low doses, nor carcinogenic. It may even prevent and treat Alzheimer's, treat certain types of epilepsy and improve symptoms of ADHD, depression and OCD. It is known to reduce rates of ulcerative colitis and pre-eclampsia.

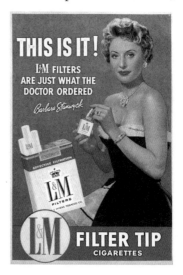

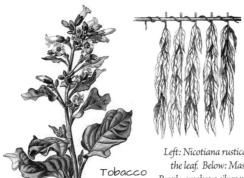

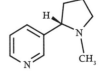

NICOTINE
$C_{10}H_{14}N_2$

Tobacco Plant

Left: Nicotiana rustica, or Aztec tobacco. Above: Drying the leaf. Below: Massasoit, leader of the Wampanoag People, smokes a silver peace pipe with governor John Carver. American shamans had smoked tobacco long before settlers brought it to 16th century Europe. By the 17th century many people were hooked, and today over one billion smoke.

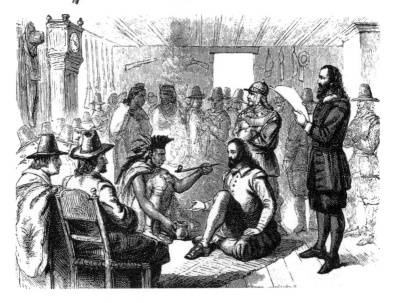

CANNABIS
peace and love

After alcohol, CANNABIS is the world's most common recreational drug. Many of the psychoactive CANNABINOID compounds are produced in the trichomes, sticky resinous buds on the female plant's flowers (*see opposite*).

There are over 400 psychoactive chemicals in cannabis. DELTA-9 TETRAHYDROCANIBINOL (THC) produces stimulating 'psychedelic' mental effects while CANNABIDIOL (CBD) provides more relaxing 'body' feelings. The overall euphoriant effect can decrease anxiety and improve sociability.

During cannabis use there is a decrease in blood flow in the brain to the *anterior insula*, *dorsomedial thalamus* and *striatum*, reducing saliency detection (the ability to tell whether what you're looking at is important). Decreased activity in the *dorsolateral prefrontal cortex* can also impair the ability to make decisions based on risk calculations. The high lasts for several hours, with music seeming more vivid, spatial perception distorted and time appearing to pass faster, accompanied by impaired cognitive and psychomotor performance, slowed reactions and short-term memory loss.

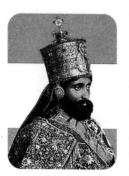
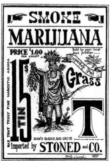
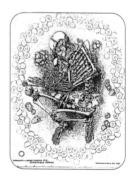

CANNABIDIOL   TETRAHYDROCANNABINOL

CBD

$C_{21}H_{30}O_2$

THC

$C_{21}H_{30}O_2$

Above: **CBD** *and* **THC**. *Cannabis has been used to treat nausea in chemotherapy, as well as symptoms of multiple sclerosis, cerebral palsy and spinal injuries. It can also help with insomnia, anxiety, depression, epilepsy, Tourette Syndrome, PTSD, dementia, diabetes and tumor growth. Alongside the THC and CBD are many other hundreds of terpenes and flavonoids that give different cannabis preparations their myriad of tastes, colours and smells.*

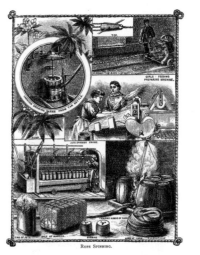

ROPE SPINNING.

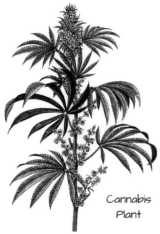

Cannabis Plant

Above: **Hemp** *rope production. In the 19th century, cannabis,* **CANNABIS SATIVA**, *was used as an anticonvulsant, antiemetic and hypnotic (Queen Victoria used it to soothe period pains). It appears in ancient Chinese culture, early Hinduism and is the "peace-giver" to Sikhs. It was revered in Germanic culture and associated with the Norse goddess, Freya. It has been used by the Islamic Sufis and is a sacrament for Rastafarians (Haile Selassie, far left). Facing page: Neolithic burial with hemp seeds.*

SOLVENTS & INHALANTS
from marker pens to sniffing poo

Inhaling solvents is a dangerous way to get high. They tend to produce a brief but intense period of extreme disorientation, euphoria and dizziness, invariably followed by a crashing headache.

There is a vast range of readily available commercial chemicals, such a paint thinners, permanent markers and glues (TOLUENE), nail polish remover (ACETONE) and aerosol gasses (CHLOROFLUROCARBONS) that produce these intoxicating effects when directly inhaled through the nose or mouth. Risks include sudden powerful palpitations, *hypoxia* (lack of oxygen), cardiac arrest and aspiration of vomit. Not to mention long-term brain damage, potential liver damage and carcinogen risks.

Kids not content with the gentle wooziness of sniffing Tipex thinners or marker pens can move on up to solvent glues. Typically the glue (such as Evo-Stick or rubber cement) is poured into a plastic bag, and the fumes inhaled, referred to as 'sniffing glue' or 'huffing'. Some solvents used in this way can produce profound hallucinations, which may or may not be considered a viable technique to glimpse the numinous. But this needs to be balanced against the unpleasant mouth sores.

JENKEM (*opposite*) is another story.

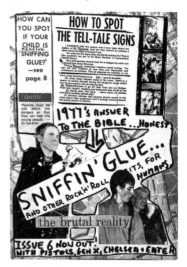

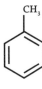
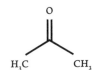
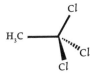

TOLUENE
C_7H_8

ACETONE
C_3H_6O

1,1,1-TRICHLOROETHANE
$C_2H_3Cl_3$

Above: Popular inhalants. Propellant gasses, such as **BUTANE** *(lighter fuel gas) have also been used. When this is propelled into the throat the resulting high is accompanied by laryngospasm as the throat rapidly cools to -20°, which can cause 'Sudden Sniffing Death Syndrome'. Keep away from flames!*

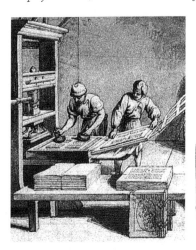

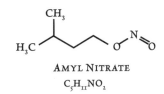

AMYL NITRATE
$C_5H_{11}NO_2$

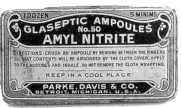

Above: **ACETONE** *was used as an ink solvent by early printers who must have got quite dizzy.* **JENKEM**, *a 1990s fad, originated amongst Zambian street children, who would take human faecal waste, ferment it for a week, and then sniff the fumes to experience brief hallucinations.*

Above: **POPPERS** (**ALKYL NITRITES**) *were sold in the 19th century to reduce the pain of cardiac angina and get high. Popular in the disco and gay scene in the 1970s, they have been used to facilitate sex, as the increasing blood flow produces a sudden relaxing of the sphincter.*

Ketamine & Nitrous Oxide
the dissociative anaesthetics

The **Dissociative Anaesthetics** have a special place in the arena of non-ordinary states of consciousness. They work by inhibition of the N-Methyl-D-aspartate (NMDA) receptor in nerve cells. When used at high doses, these drugs can induce total anaesthesia, while at lower doses they produce marked psychedelic effects, including a trance-like sensation of dreamy out-of-body hallucinatory detachment from one's surroundings.

Nitrous oxide has a long history in medicine and culture. Also referred to as **Laughing Gas**, it has assisted dentists and enthralled users for over a century. When inhaled from a balloon, the user experiences a brief moment of light-headedness and spacy psychedelic wonder, often accompanied by interesting phaser-like distortions of sound.

Phencyclidine, also known as **PCP** or **Angel Dust**, was a precursor to **Ketamine** which is still widely used in human medicine as a short-acting anaesthetic. Perfect for replacing shoulder dislocations, it is much safer and more convenient that dosing patients up with gallons of benzodiazepines and opiates that then require an overnight stay in hospital.

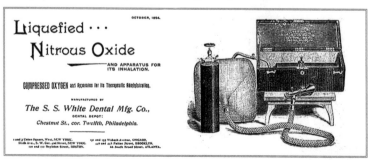

PHENCYCLIDINE

$C_{17}H_{25}N$

KETAMINE

$C_{13}H_{16}ClNO$

$$N \equiv \overset{+}{N} - O^- \longleftrightarrow {}^-N = \overset{+}{N} = O$$

NITROUS OXIDE

N_2O

*Left: **PCP**, or **ANGEL DUST**, was a 1950s & 1960s anaesthetic which became a recreational drug in the 1970s in the US. It was replaced by **KETAMINE**, which is popular for to its hallucinatory effects and may have promise as a treatment for depression. If used excessively it becomes addictive and causes irreversible damage to the urinary tract, leading to bladder removal and urostomy bags. Ketamine works in the brain to modulate levels of glutamate and GABA (see p.6), which can affect levels of anxiety and depression.*

*Below: First synthesised in 1772 by Joseph Priestly, **NITROUS OXIDE** was popularised by Humphry Davy, later president of the Royal Society, who named it "Laughing Gas". It was used for seduction and euphoria at parties in the 1800s and only as an anaesthetic from 1844. Today it is popular at festivals where it is sold in balloons.*

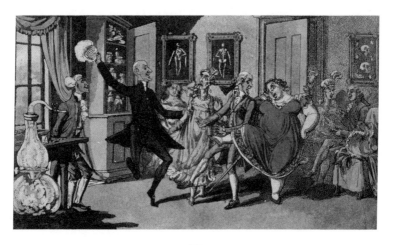

COCAINE

green leaves and white lines

COCAINE, a crystalline psychoactive alkaloid from the leaves of the COCA plant, is a strong stimulant and appetite suppressant. Although very psychologically addictive, it rarely induces physical dependency.

Cocaine use increases levels of dopamine (*see p.6*) between nerve cells by preventing its reuptake. In the brain's reward centre, this reinforces behaviour, resulting in the desire to re-dose. Over time tolerance develops, requiring the user to take larger and more frequent doses to feel the same high or to avoid withdrawal. Overdose can cause death by heart attack.

South Americans have been chewing coca leaves (with a pinch of lime) for thousands of years for health and longevity (*see opposite*). However, cocaine in its purified powdered form is considerably stronger. By the turn of the 20th century it was everywhere, recognised as an effective restorative for many ills. Shackleton took it to Antarctica, Scott carried it to the South Pole, Sigmund Freud extolled its virtues and a glass of Coca-Cola once contained just under 10 milligrams. In the 1980s, the intense freebase form of cocaine, CRACK, ravaged American inner city ghettos. By the 1990s cocaine was the second most prevalent illegal drug in the world behind cannabis.

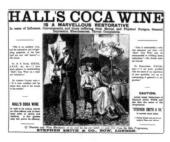

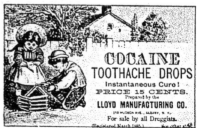

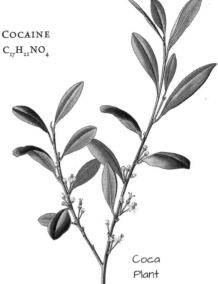

COCAINE
$C_{17}H_{21}NO_4$

Above: **COCAINE**, *benzoylmethyl ecgonine, is a tropane alkaloid, which is weakly alkaline and reacts with acids to form salts. Cocaine hydrochloride is the most often encountered form. There are no simple substitution treatments for dependency as there are for opiates; users are instead engaged in psychosocial interventions. Cocaine abuse is highly destructive.*

Coca
Plant

Above: **THE COCA PLANT** *has been cultivated since at least 6000 BC in northern Peru. The Inca chewed the leaves to alleviate hunger and thirst while working. Today the plant is grown as a cash crop in Bolivia, Columbia, Ecuador and Peru for the extraction of cocaine.*

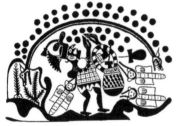

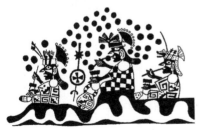

Left: Paintings from a Moche jar, Chimu, Peru, c.500AD. The Conquistadors demonised chewing coca leaves, but instead of eradicating it they taxed it. By the late 19th century even the pope had a taste for **MARIANI WINE**, *which, along with other tonic wines, contained significant amounts of cocaine.*

OPIATES
from Xanadu to rehab

Derived from the heads of the **PAPAVER SOMNIFERUM** poppy (*opposite*), the **OPIATES** are among the most intriguing, misunderstood and useful substances on the planet, and alas also some of the most dangerous. They give an altered state like a heavy blanket of euphoria, tapping into our desire for ultimate contentment. Medicinally, the healing analgesic effects of opium have been widely used to relieve pain since Neolithic times.

Naturally occurring opiates include **CODEINE** and **MORPHINE**. **SYNTHETIC OPIOIDS** are synthesised drugs with opiate-like effects, examples being **FENTANYL** (which is 50–100 times stronger than morphine), **PETHIDINE** (used as an analgesic during childbirth) and **BUPRENORPHINE** (a safer alternative to methadone, used in opioid substitution therapy).

Opiates mimic the body's naturally produced endorphins, binding easily to our endogenous opioid receptors and acting directly on the central nervous system. Endorphins are generally released in response to pleasure (e.g. during sex, as a reward) or pain (e.g. during exercise, to reduce pain). As a result, the potential for psychological addiction to these drugs is intense.

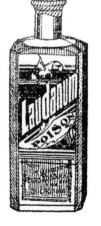

Prolonged use of opiates, of which **DIAMORPHINE** (**HEROIN**) is the most powerful, can lead to extreme physical dependence (e.g. in 1905 around 25% of Chinese men were users). Heavy users face a painful withdrawal if they are not taken on a daily basis. For some, dependence can lead to a severely maladaptive destructive lifestyle.

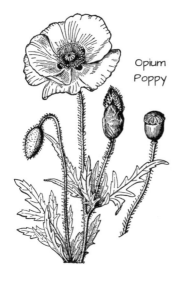

Opium Poppy

MORPHINE

$C_{17}H_{19}NO_3$

H$_3$C

FENTANYL

$C_{22}H_{28}N_2O$

Above and below: The Opium Poppy has been harvested since at least 4500 BC. Shallow cuts are scored into the unripe pods. These bleed milky tears which dry to a sticky brown resin.

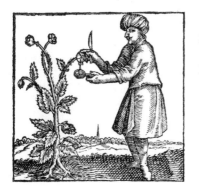

Above: In the early 19th century the active component MORPHINE (named after the Greek god of sleep, Morpheus) was isolated from opium and the drug became a popular tonic.

Above: FENTANYL, a synthetic opiod, is used for pain relief. It has been notoriously over-prescribed by doctors. Extremely potent, it often harms street heroin users when sold as heroin.

Facing page: LAUDANUM was a popular drug in the 19th century and is still available today. An opium tincture containing 10% opium by weight (the equivalent of 1% morphine), it was cheaper than gin or wine. The Romantic poets and the pre-Raphaelite painters were all addicted to it, as was Abraham Lincoln's wife. Samuel Taylor Coleridge's wrote his epic poem Kubla Khan, during a laudanum experience.

MDMA & AMPHETAMINES
khat and other stimulants

Many natural stimulants give a little lift—plants like GURUANA, COFFEE (*see page 28*) and KHAT (*below*). The synthetic stimulant AMPHETAMINE (or SPEED) was first synthesised in 1887 and produces a mildly zoomed up feeling. Consumption leads to increased heart rate, raised blood pressure, tremors and sweats, as well as hyperactivity, insomnia, reduced appetite, rapid speech, racing thoughts and increased levels of alertness. Its much stronger and more addictive cousin is METHAMPHETAMINE (*see opposite*).

Another cousin, 3,4-methylenedioxymethamphetamine (MDMA or ECSTASY) is widely used recreationally but is also useful in psychotherapy due to its remarkable qualities (*see opposite*). It reduces depression, increases closeness and raises arousal, whilst paradoxically promoting relaxation and new solutions to old problems. When taken under favourable conditions the experience is pleasurable to almost every user, almost every time.

Chewing KHAT leaves (*below*) has been part of North African and Arab culture for thousands of years. Its mild stimulant, CATHINONE, gives users a gentle coffee-like buzz. More recently, khat made headlines because of a concentrated semi-synthetic form of cathinone, METHYLCATHINONE, (M-CAT, MEOW MEOW or MEPHEDRONE). Mephedrone is to khat what cocaine is to coca, a far stronger stimulant which has a rushy high with a severe comedown. Users can easily become dependent and often report using the drug for many days and nights in a row.

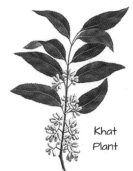

Khat Plant

MDMA $C_{11}H_{15}NO_2$

CATHINONE $C_9H_{11}NO$

AMPHETAMINE $C_9H_{13}N$

METHAMPHETAMINE $C_{10}H_{15}N$

*Above: Popular amphetamines. **METHAMPHETAMINE** or **CRYSTAL METH** or **ICE** is the racemic free base equal mixture of **LEVOMETHAMPHETAMINE** and **DEXTROMETHAMPHETAMINE** in their pure amine forms. Meth users experience a rapidly elevated mood, increased alertness, concentration and energy, and reduced appetite. At high doses, it is associated with psychosis and significant physical harms.*

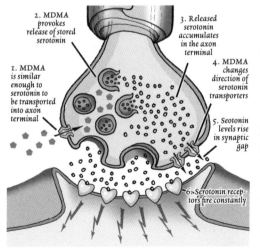

2. MDMA provokes release of stored serotonin

1. MDMA is similar enough to serotonin to be transported into axon terminal

3. Released serotonin accumulates in the axon terminal

4. MDMA changes direction of serotonin transporters

5. Serotonin levels rise in synaptic gap

6. Serotonin receptors fire constantly

*Left: **MDMA** or **ECSTASY** or **MOLLY** precipitates a massive release of stored serotonin from vesicles in the pre-synaptic membrane. This floods the synaptic gap and transmits nerve impulses to the post-synaptic neurotransmitters. Popular on the dance scene, the pleasurable effects begin 30–45 mins after taking the drug and last for 3–6 hours. Adverse effects include teeth grinding, rapid heartbeat, sweating and dehydration, blurred vision, difficulty sleeping and ensuing depression and fatigue.*

NATURAL PSYCHEDELICS
psilocybin, DMT *and mescaline*

The 'classic' psychedelics are the three shown here plus LSD (*overleaf*). Thought to be partial agonists at serotonin 2A receptors in the pyramidal cells of layer V of the cerebral cortex, they produce temporary psychological, visual and auditory effects and an altered state of consciousness.

PSILOCYBIN occurs in many 'magic' mushrooms, including *Psilocybe Cyanescens, Psilocybe mexicana, Psilocybe azurescens* and *Psilocybe semilanceata* (*illustrated below*) which may be eaten raw, dried or brewed as a tea. Psilocybin is relatively safe with a lethal dose being over 1000 times that needed for intoxication. The effects last for 2–6 hours, though seem to last longer.

MESCALINE is found in a number of cacti, particularly PEYOTE and SAN PEDRO, and has been used since time immemorial in Native American ceremonies. Peyote has a bitter taste and the strong psychedelic effects can last over 12 hours. One side effect is nausea, although if you are glimpsing the secrets of the universe you may not be so worried about throwing up.

DIMETHYLTRYPTAMINE or DMT occurs naturally in a form that normally has no effect on humans when taken orally. However, when smoked or injected it produces an intense, short-lived experience. It is an active ingredient in the South American shamanic brew AYAHUASCA.

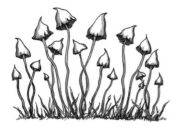

PSILOCYBIN
$C_{12}H_{17}N_2O_4P$

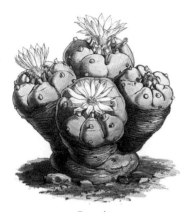

Peyote
Cactus

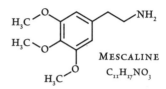

MESCALINE

$C_{11}H_{17}NO_3$

Left: The **PEYOTE CACTUS**, *Lophophora Williamsii*. Aldous Huxley's experience with mescaline in 1953 led him to write The Doors of Perception, *catapulting him into psychedelic culture. The title was taken from William Blake's 1794* Marriage of Heaven and Hell:

"If the doors of perception were cleansed every thing would appear to man as it is: Infinite. For man has closed himself up, till he sees all things thro' narrow chinks of his cavern."

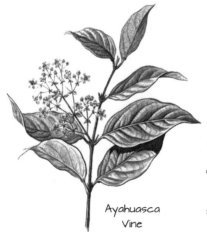

Ayahuasca
Vine

DMT

$C_{12}H_{16}N_2$

Left: **AYAHUASCA VINE**. *DMT produces significant effects on the electrical activity of the brain, with a very strong reduction of alpha waves, which normally appear when the eyes are closed. The intense otherworldliness of DMT, and the chemical resemblance to serotonin has lead some to wonder whether spontaneous mystical experiences could actually be mediated by a release of endogenous DMT.*

LSD

and the psychedelic experience

LSD, or **ACID**, is a semi-synthetic compound, derived from the **ERGOT** fungus that grows on **RYE**. Incredibly potent, it is active at a dose of 25 millionths of a gram, yet is virtually physiologically inert, with physical overdose practically unheard of. For many, the LSD experience is an encounter with a wider awareness than the usual boundaries of self allow.

LSD binds to most serotonin receptor subtypes, but its psychedelic effects are likely attributed primarily to the 5-HT2A subtype. An associated probable mechanism of action of psychedelic effects is related to an increase in glutamate release in the cerebral cortex.

LSD has been described as a 'non-specific amplifier', such that any emotion, benign or destructive, can be magnified to dramatic proportions. A frequent effect is the heightening or distortion of perceptions in all the senses. Sounds become vivid, vision flows as if alive and colours appear brighter. Time may move forwards, backwards or freeze. There may be fluctuating thoughts and emotions, death-rebirth phenomena and a sense of feeling close to and understanding others' points of view.

There are strong links between psychedelics and meditation. In the 1960s George Harrison and other philosophical users of LSD travelled to India to learn meditation as a means to continue exploring the psychological and spiritual realms they had initially unlocked with drugs.

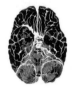

PLACEBO

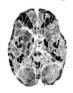 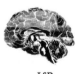

LSD

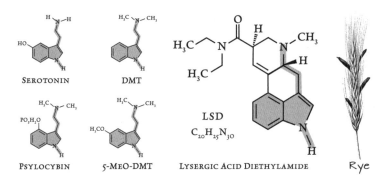

Above: The neurotransmitter SEROTONIN *shares a core* INDOLEAMINE *structure (shaded) with several psychedelics, including* LSD, *although even small variations in chemical structure can lead to very different psychological effects.* *Right:* The ERGOT *fungus (darker grains) which grows on* RYE, *contains* LYSERGIC ACID, *a precursor for the synthesis of LSD. Careful use of LSD can be beneficial, although the philosopher Alan Watts said about its repeated use, "Once you get the message, hang up the phone."*

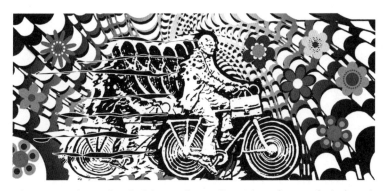

Above: LSD was discovered accidently by Swiss chemist Albert Hofmann [1906-2008], who famously self-dosed on 19th April 1943 with 250 micrograms, thinking it would be undetectable (it is in fact a most righteous trip). Psychonauts still commemorate this date as 'Bicycle Day,' celebrating Hofmann's ride home from his laboratory in a profoundly altered state of consciousness: "I had wonderful visions ... was completely astonished by the beauty of nature ... the intense play of colours and forms ..." etc.

Poisons & Potions
bewitching botanics

Altered states are as old as the hills. The Romans enjoyed WINE (*p.30*), OPIUM (*p.42*), CANNABIS (*p.34*) and DATURA (*opposite*). However, with the rise of Christianity in Europe, psychedelic states were demonised, along with the knowledge of the herbs, roots, flowers and fungi to create them. Yet, throughout the Middle Ages people still sought them out.

The alkaloids in HENBANE and MANDRAKE produce hallucinations. BELLADONNA (DEADLY NIGHTSHADE) has high concentrations of ATROPINE, which causes a powerful anticholinergic reaction of blurred vision, dilated pupils and tachycardia, plus a dreamy delirium. Closely related DATURA (also known as JIMSON WEED, DEVIL'S APPLE or THORN APPLE) contains SCOPOLAMINE, ATROPINE and HYOSCAMINE, which cause disorientation and hallucinations. Medieval witches used it as 'flying ointment', and it is still used by shamans in India and Africa.

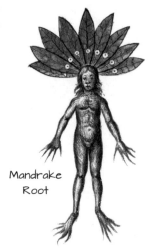

Mandrake Root

Today, a whole pharmacopeia of amazing plants and fungi are used across the world in a spiritual context. Examples include the shamanic use of SALVIA DIVINORUM in Mexico, COHOBA in the Caribbean, AYAHUASCA in South America, KAVA from Pacific Polynesia, KRATOM (MAMBOG) in South East Asia, South African SCELETIUM (MESEMBRYANTHEMUM or CHANNA) and the Xhosa visionary plant medicine UBULAWU (DREAM ROOT).

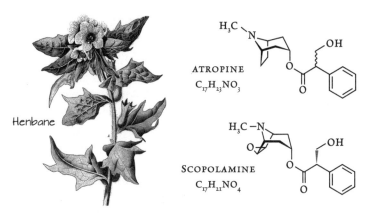

Henbane

ATROPINE
$C_{17}H_{23}NO_3$

SCOPOLAMINE
$C_{17}H_{21}NO_4$

Three plants from the the **SOLANACEAE** *family. Above left:* **BLACK HENBANE** *or Stinking Nightshade. Below left:* **BELLADONNA** *or Deadly Nightshade. Below right:* **DATURA** *or Devil's Trumpet. Above right: Hallucinogenic atropine and scopolamine molecules. Facing page: The* **MANDRAKE** *root.*

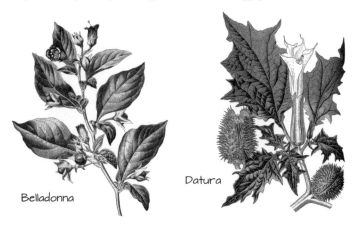

Belladonna

Datura

Another option is **CANE TOAD LICKING**. *The toad is not actually licked, the parotid gland behind the animal's ear is milked to produce a substance rich in 5-MEO-DMT and bufotenin. When dried and smoked it produces a high similar to that of LSD or psilocybin (the toad is unharmed by the practice).*

SHAMANISM
healing hallucinogens

Psychoactive plants and fungi have been used by shamans for a very long time. Around 5,000 years ago, early Indo-Iranians were purportedly drinking a magical potion called SOMA. Mentioned in the *Rig Vedas* (ancient Sanskrit texts that form the basis of the Hindu and Zoroastrian traditions), this mystery substance allowed direct communication with the gods.

The ancient Greeks were also keen hallucinogen users. The Eleusinian Rites were practiced annually for over 2,000 years to worship the goddesses Demeter and Persephone. After fasting, initiates drank a special brew, the KYKEON, before entering the Telestrion Hall. Here they experienced mysterious visions and gained knowledge of life after death. What was the kykeon? Perhaps it was DALLIS GRASS (*below*), impregnated with ERGOT fungus (*see page 49*), or opium or some type of psychedelic mushroom.

In the frozen wastes of Siberia shamans still search the bases of
pine, spruce, birch and cedar trees for that
classic red toadstool with white spots, the
AMANITA MUSCARIA mushroom. It contains
MUSCIMOL and IBOTENIC ACID, whose
cholinergic effects cause nausea, drowsiness
and low blood pressure, but also a marked
psychedelic effect when prepared and taken
correctly. Reindeer go to great lengths to
seek out and eat amanita, and shamans collect
and drink their urine as a safe way of taking
the drug, as the urine contains virtually
unchanged muscimol.

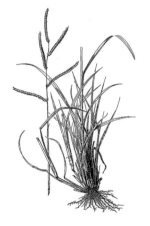

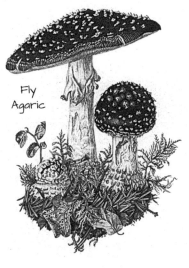

Fly Agaric

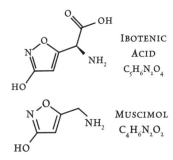

IBOTENIC ACID
$C_5H_6N_2O_4$

MUSCIMOL
$C_4H_6N_2O_2$

Left: The classic red- and white-spotted
AMANITA MUSCARIA *or* **FLY AGARIC** *toadstool*
contains **IBOTENIC ACID** *and* **MUSCIMOL**.
Many images of Christmas (red and white
livery, flying reindeer and pine trees) arise from
Siberian shamanic links to Amanita muscaria.

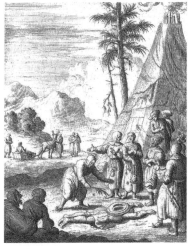

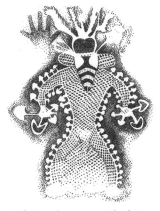

Left: Lappish ceremony, Finland, 1682.
Above: The Algerian Tassili mushroom
shaman rock painting, dated to c.8000 BC.

ANTIDEPRESSANTS
the search for the magic pill

Underlying the industry of modern antidepressant therapy are a number of questionable 'biological models'. The *Monoamine Hypothesis* proposes that monoamine neurotransmitters, such as serotonin, norepinephrine, dopamine and epinephrine are deficient in people with depression. In the 1950s, the TRICYCLIC ANTIDEPRESSANTS, such as AMITRIPTYLINE, CLOMIPRAMINE and IMIPRAMINE, were used to bluntly block the synaptic reuptake of monoamines, thus keeping them available. But these drugs came with a host of side effects, particularly associated cardiac risks.

Then came the rise of the *Selective Serotonin Reuptake Inhibitors* (SSRIs), which block serotonin reuptake (FLUOXETINE or PROZAC, CITALOPRAM, SERTRALINE and PAROXETINE). These did reduce the cardiac side effects.

There then followed a host of other specific reuptake blockers to target the other monoamines: SNRIs which block serotonin and norepinephrine (VENLAFAXINE, TRAMADOL and DULOXETINE), SARIs which antagonise serotonin receptors and inhibit the reuptake of serotonin, norepinephrine, or dopamine (TRAZODONE and NEFAZODONE) and many more besides.

In the future, psychedelic-assisted psychotherapy may actually begin get to the heart of people's problems and help address the causes of their depression, rather than just the symptoms.

TRAZODONE
$C_{19}H_{22}ClN_5O$

FLUOXETINE
$C_{17}H_{18}F_3NO$

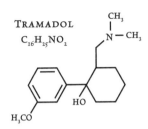

AMITRIPTYLINE
$C_{20}H_{23}N$

TRAMADOL
$C_{16}H_{25}NO_2$

Below: Sorrowing Old Man, Vincent Van Gogh, 1890. Depression and anxiety are hugely complex emotional states tied up intimately with a person's genetics, their childhood, their history of attachment and parenting, their schooling, living circumstances, education, employment status and a host of other psychosocial factors.

This page and opposite: Popular antidepressant pills seek to 'rescue a human being from their many complex influences, past and present, and brighten their future'. The pharmaceutical industry dishes out this dream in the form of happy pills, designed to be taken daily for decades, as 'maintenance therapy'.

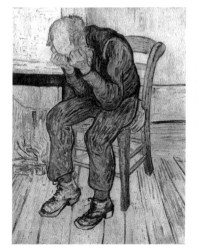

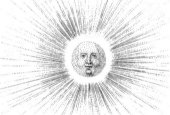

Remember: Daily antidepressants a) Only target the symptoms of depression, and are not a cure. b) Are not especially effective in cases of low to moderate depression. c) Take up to six weeks to start working. d) Are not free of side effects. e) Have a nasty withdrawal syndrome when attempting to come off them. f) Have been widely over-prescribed in primary care.

Quantum Consciousness
beyond the brain

Modern science struggles to explain consciousness. Some intensely altered states feel like being connected with everything everywhere. Is this a confused illusion, or a revelation of consciousness as it truly is? Perhaps quantum phenomena such as entanglement and superposition play a role.

Plato proposed the concept of PANPSYCHISM, that mind exists outside the brain. Perhaps the brain does not create consciousness (or even the illusion of it), but rather acts as a lens to focus some more universal awareness.

BIOCENTRISM goes further, with the belief that life is fundamental and that consciousness created the universe, not the other way around. The implication is that intelligence may have existed prior to matter, and that space and time are but tools of our animal understanding.

In the 1950s and 1960s tens of thousands of patients were effectively treated with LSD and other psychedelic drugs. These became demonised for socio-political reasons, and almost all research was halted for the next forty years, but psychedelics are now being investigated again. LSD, psilocybin and the entactogen MDMA are all safe physiologically at therapeutic dosages, have a low dependency risk and can be used effectively as adjuncts to psychotherapy for patients with a range of psychiatric disorders.

The 'War On Drugs' has failed to reduce the use of drugs, the misuse of drugs, the health risks posed by drugs and the criminality associated with the misuse of drugs. Maybe one day we will be able to go into a specialised drug treatment centre on any high street and be provided with a safe, monitored and effective altered state experience for personal growth and spiritual development. Until then, we will no doubt see many more people taking risks and settling for those green potatoes. Stay safe.

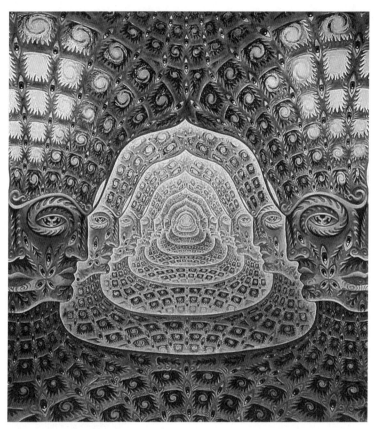

Above: DMT (detail) by Alex Grey. A vision of the universe as mind, and mind as the universe. Literature about the use of psychedelics, particularly DMT, is full of imagery describing pan-universal communications with other levels of reality and associated beings. Some writers believe psychedelics act as doorways to interdimensional travel and facilitate connection with a panpsychic consciousness. Across the aeons, countless drug-assisted developmental sessions have taken place, each in a suitable setting accompanied by close supervision from a shaman or therapist with whom the patient has built up a trusting therapeutic bond before taking the substance. This is a part of our human heritage.

FURTHER READING

There are heaps of books, academic papers and journals, from the 1950s to the present day, about the subject of altered states of consciousness and particularly psychedelic drugs. Some useful texts are listed below, along with a few links to contemporary research groups exploring this subject.

Doblin, Rick and Burge, Brad, (editors.) *Manifesting Minds: A Review of Psychedelics in Science, Medicine, Sex, and Spirituality* (2014). Evolver Editions, Berkeley, CA, USA.

Fadiman, J. *The Psychedelic Explorer's Guide: Safe, therapeutic, and sacred journeys* (2011). Park Street Press, Rochester, Vermont.

Grinspoon, Lester. and Bakalar, J. (1979) *Psychedelic Drugs Reconsidered*. The Lindesmith Center, New York.

Grof, Stanislav. *LSD Psychotherapy* (3rd ed.) (2001). MAPS, Sarasota.

Hofmann, A. *LSD My Problem Child: Reflections on Sacred Drugs, Mysticism, and Science* (1979 / 2005). MAPS, Sarasota.

Holland, Julie (editor) *Ecstasy: The Complete Guide: A Comprehensive Look at the Risks and Benefits of MDMA* (2001/2010). Park Street Press, New York.

Huxley, Aldous. (Edited by Michael Horowitz and Cynthia Palmer). *Moksha: Aldous Huxley's Classic Writings on Psychedelics and the Visionary Experience* (1999). Park Street Press, New York.

Leary, Timothy. *High Priest* (1968). The New American Library Inc., New York.

Letcher, Andy. *Shroom: A Cultural History of the Magic Mushroom* (2007). Ecco, London.

Masters, R.L. and Houston, J. *The Varieties of Psychedelic Experience* (1966). Park Street Press, Rochester, Vermont.

McKenna, Terence. *Food of the Gods* (1982). Bantam Press, London.

Pollan, M. *How to change your mind: What the new science of psychedelics teaches us about consciousness, dying, addiction, depression, and transcendence* (2018). Penguin Press, New York.

Roberts, Andy. *Albion Dreaming: A popular history of LSD in Britain* (2008). Marshall Cavendish, London.

Roberts, Thomas B. *Psychedelic Horizons* (2006). Imprint Academic, Charlottesville.

Sessa, B. *The Psychedelic Renaissance* (2012 / 2017). Aeon Books, London.

Strassman, Rick. *DMT: The Spirit Molecule* (2001). Park Street Press, New York.

Tart, Charles, editor. *Altered States of Consciousness* (1969). John Wiley and Sons, New York.

Winkelman, M. and Sessa, B. (editors) *Advances in Psychedelic Medicine: State-of-the-Art Therapeutic Applications*. ABC / Clio Publishers, New York.

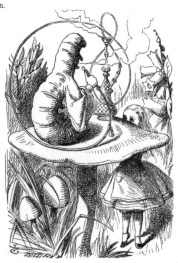

For all the latest news and published papers on consciousness research and psychedelics:

www.beckleyfoundation.org

www.erowid.org

www.maps.org

www.heffter.org

www.breakingconvention.co.uk